What Is

# Syphilis?

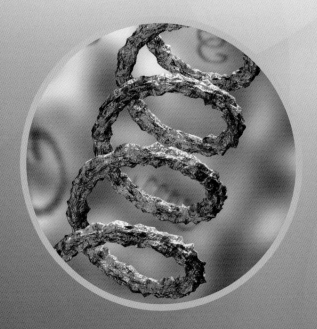

Ursula Pang

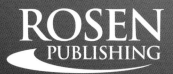
ROSEN
PUBLISHING

NEW YORK

Published in 2022 by The Rosen Publishing Group, Inc.
29 East 21st Street, New York, NY 10010

First Edition

Portions of this work were originally authored by Philip Wolny and published as *Syphilis.* All new material in this edition was authored by Ursula Pang.

Library of Congress Cataloging-in-Publication Data

Names: Pang, Ursula, author.
Title: What is syphilis? / Ursula Pang
Description: New York : Rosen Publishing, [2022] | Series: Sexual health
    awareness | Includes index.
Identifiers: LCCN 2021035646 (print) | LCCN 2021035647 (ebook) | ISBN
    9781499472288 (library binding) | ISBN 9781499472271 (paperback) | ISBN
    9781499472295 (ebook)
Subjects: LCSH: Syphilis--History. | Sexually transmitted diseases.
Classification: LCC RC201 .P22 2022  (print) | LCC RC201  (ebook) | DDC
    616.95/13--dc23
LC record available at https://lccn.loc.gov/2021035646
LC ebook record available at https://lccn.loc.gov/2021035647

Manufactured in the United States of America

Some of the images in this book illustrate individuals who are models. The depictions do not imply actual situations or events.

CPSIA Compliance Information: Batch #CWRYA22. For further information contact Rosen Publishing, New York, New York at 1-800-237-9932.

Find us on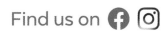

# CONTENTS

# INTRODUCTION

Syphilis may sound like a thing of the past. After all, isn't that the disease that killed mob boss Al Capone (1899–1947) and, possibly, philosopher Friedrich Nietzsche (1844–1900)? Who gets syphilis anymore? Is it something teens have to worry about today?

While today syphilis is curable in its early stages and treatable in its late stages, it's still a threat to people. When penicillin was first used to treat syphilis in the 1940s, rates began to drop dramatically in the United States. They continued dropping until around 2000

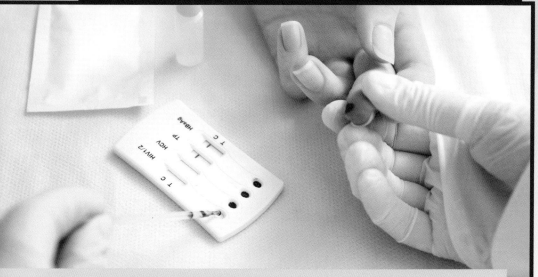

In the past, people couldn't identify syphilis until the disease was very obvious. Now, doctors can identify this infection with a simple blood test.

and 2001, but then they started to increase again. In 2018, the rate of syphilis cases hit a record high since 1991, with 115,045 cases (according to the Centers for Disease Control and Prevention, or CDC). That same year, researchers at the University of California Los Angeles reported that each year, there are 6 million new cases of syphilis worldwide in people aged 15 to 49. Complications of untreated syphilis are serious, and even more so when a person also has HIV (human immunodeficiency virus).

If syphilis is treatable, then what's the big deal? Syphilis may respond very well to penicillin, but it's also very dangerous if left untreated. It can easily be transmitted through sex—vaginal, anal, and oral— with an infected person. And while early symptoms of the disease may seem very mild or even be invisible in some people, complications arise in later stages of untreated syphilis. Throughout history, untreated syphilis led to severe disability and even death. That's still a serious threat today in places of the world without adequate health care and resources.

Syphilis isn't something many people think about when they're deciding if they're going to have sex. But it's better to consider the risks and work to prevent it than to have to deal with a positive diagnosis. If you're going to have sex, you're going to have to think about STIs (sexually transmitted infections), which can turn into STDs (sexually transmitted diseases). This might seem like a downer, but knowledge gives you the power to keep yourself and your partner safe from illness.

If you do contract syphilis, it's not the end of the

world, but it does need to be taken seriously. It really pays to muster the courage to confront a possible infection head on. Some people ignore it, hoping it goes away. But delaying diagnosis and treatment only gives syphilis a chance to cause more damage to your body and infect other people.

STDs, including syphilis, don't only cause physical symptoms and suffering. They can also cause embarrassment, anger, anxiety, and depression. Coping with an STD requires attention to your mental and emotional well-being, a strong support system, and self-care. Socially, STDs may cause embarrassment and shame, leading people to hide their infections.

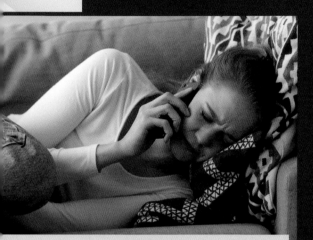

Getting the news that you have an STD can be really hard. Having strong coping skills can help you get through difficult moments.

Syphilis can affect people of any sexual orientation and gender identity. However, it's important to know how STDs can affect you based on your assigned sex at birth (a label based on your hormones, chromosomes, and genitals at birth) or the body parts you have. Although it might feel wrong to think of yourself with that assigned label, those genetic, hormonal, and anatomical factors play a role in how STDs affect you. For example, biological males contract syphilis at a higher rate than biological females. However, biological females have a different concern—if they're pregnant while having syphilis, they could suffer a miscarriage or stillbirth, or they could have a baby with congenital syphilis.

You can arm yourself with the greatest protection against syphilis—knowledge. The more you know, the more you can be empowered to make the right choices for you. You can understand how to prevent syphilis and how to recognize its symptoms. You can learn how to get tested and deal with a positive diagnosis. Hopefully one day, with education and medicine, syphilis can truly be a disease of the past.

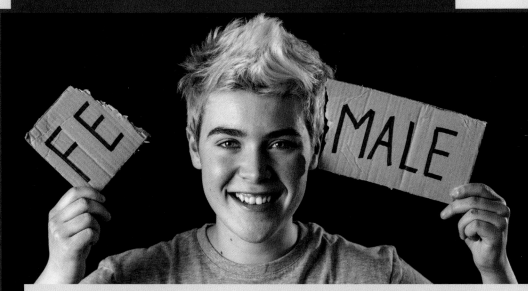

For transgender people who are transitioning through hormone therapy or surgery, it's important to understand the ways in which specific STDs can affect your body.

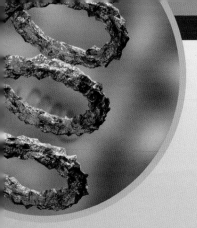

## CHAPTER 1

# SYPHILIS MAKES A COMEBACK

**B**acteria exists everywhere in the world and everywhere in our bodies. These tiny microorganisms can only be seen with magnifying tools such as microscopes. Some bacteria are beneficial, such as good bacteria in the gut that helps you digest food. Other bacteria can be harmful or even deadly.

Harmful bacteria can lead to major health problems, and even death. *Treponema pallidum* is a spirochete—a long, thin, coiled bacterium. It can harm several organ systems, and it can be fatal if left unchecked. We can take a look throughout history to see how this bacterium has affected people around the world—and how it poses a threat today.

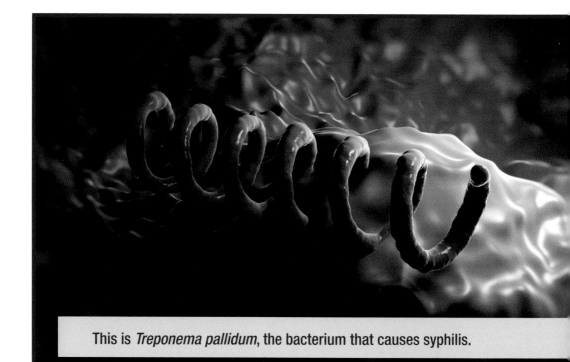

This is *Treponema pallidum*, the bacterium that causes syphilis.

## SYPHILIS IN HISTORY

It's hard to track the origins of syphilis. That's because the symptoms have been mistaken for other diseases such as leprosy. Syphilis has probably existed for thousands of years in different parts of the globe. There's evidence to suggest that the sexually transmitted form of syphilis can be traced back to 3000 BC in Southwest Asia. It likely grew in strength and virulence throughout time as it migrated with human populations. Another theory is that syphilis originated in the New World and was brought back to Europe by explorers. Some of its symptoms among Europeans may have been confused with those of leprosy, which has similar effects as late-stage syphilis. Artwork and writings from both the Western and Eastern Hemispheres can give researchers clues into how syphilis may have developed and migrated.

By the 16th century, syphilis was widespread in Europe. Because medical knowledge was far more primitive, its late-stage symptoms were even more devastating to sufferers then. Syphilis thus gained its fearsome reputation. It also became a political issue. As it spread, neighboring countries and different religions

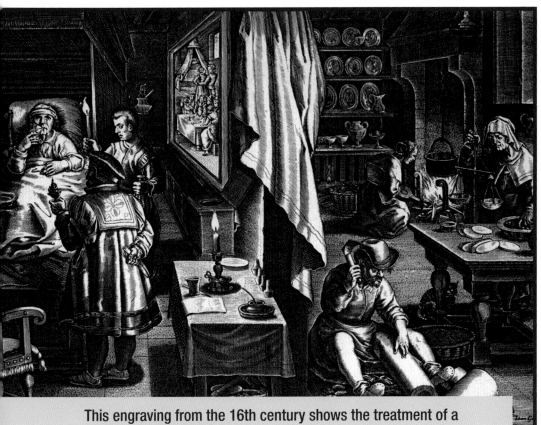

This engraving from the 16th century shows the treatment of a syphilis patient in Europe.

would blame one another for the disease. People who lived in today's Poland called it "the German Disease," while the Turks called it "the Christian disease." People in today's Italy, Germany, and the United Kingdom called it "the French disease." In India, Muslims and Hindus blamed one another for syphilis. The stigma around the disease was one of its defining features.

## STORIES OF FAME AND SYPHILIS

Throughout history, many famous figures have been said to have syphilis. Some people believe the famous author Oscar Wilde (1854–1900) died from late-stage syphilis. Al Capone, Prohibition-era mob boss of the Chicago Outfit, survived violent gang life and a long prison sentence in Alcatraz but may have died of syphilis. Famous painters Paul Gaugin (1848–1903) and Édouard Manet (1832–1883) also suffered and died from syphilis. It's even rumored that Nazi dictator Adolf Hitler (1889–1945) had neurosyphilis, which caused intense mood swings and added to his motivation to systematically murder Jewish people, whom he blamed for spreading what he saw as a "Jewish disease."

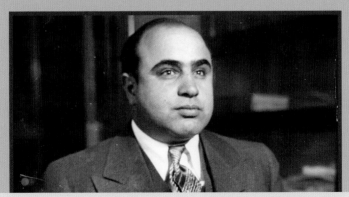

Al Capone was serving a sentence at Alcatraz federal prison when his syphilis became serious. This illness eventually got him out of jail, so he could serve out his sentence at home.

Wars are often great opportunities for STDs to spread, and syphilis is no exception. That's because there's movement of many people from one place to another. Ports and seaside cities often became hotbeds of STD transmission as soldiers found comfort in brothels. While an STD like gonorrhea might cause immediate symptoms and discomfort, syphilis is a long-lasting disease with symptoms that seem mild or latent for months or years. Over 73,000 Union soldiers were treated for syphilis during the American Civil War. World War I presented an even greater challenge; a worldwide war meant more exposure to disease. While the French military gave their soldiers condoms to stay safe from STDs, the U.S. military preached abstinence and saw great numbers of STDs. More than 350,000 U.S. soldiers were reported sick with syphilis and gonorrhea during World War I.

In the United States, syphilis cases hit a peak of about 106,000 in 1947, according to the U.S. Centers for Disease Control and Prevention (CDC). The widespread use of penicillin then helped reduce its spread greatly. Scientists declared the disease almost eradicated in North America around 2000, but it has since rebounded. Meanwhile, in the developing world, millions are infected annually. Because it was seen as nearly eradicated, and because the disease takes a long time to cause great discomfort, people often don't take syphilis seriously. For many people in the United States, it seems like a problem of the past. Unfortunately, that's far from the truth.

## THE TUSKEGEE SYPHILIS STUDY

Between 1932 and 1972, the U.S. Public Health Service conducted a clinical study in Tuskegee, Alabama. This immoral and irresponsible study observed the natural history of untreated syphilis. The participants were mainly Black Americans, who were told they were being treated for "bad blood." The researchers didn't collect informed consent from participants, nor did they offer treatment for syphilis after penicillin was available and proven to treat the disease. They allowed the disease to spread and advance in the people they were studying, so that they could see the effects of the disease on the human body. Since 1972, ethical standards for studies have gotten better because of what happened in Tuskegee, and in 1997, President Bill Clinton issued a formal apology. However, the injustices and deep wounds suffered by the Tuskegee men and their families are long lasting. Even today, some Black Americans find it hard to trust medical professionals because of inequities in health care and studies like this one that didn't treat Black people with respect or human decency.

## PENICILLIN TO THE RESCUE

Treatments for syphilis throughout history were unhelpful and sometimes even toxic or deadly. Before the 20th century, thousands of people died annually when their syphilis infections were treated with toxic substances, including mercury and arsenic. The antibiotic penicillin had few comparable side effects. Along with syphilis, it fought dozens of other ailments, earning the nickname "the wonder drug."

In 1943, doctors at the U.S. Marine Hospital on Staten Island, New York, cured four patients of syphilis within eight days. This helped the military, which was fighting in World War II. Prior to that, syphilis, gonorrhea, and other STDs took many soldiers out of work, sometimes for months at a time. The need to produce large amounts of penicillin quickly to give to many thousands of troops would translate to mass-producing it for civilian uses after the war too.

Today, penicillin is still used to treat syphilis. It can cure syphilis but can't undo damage already caused by the infection. That's why it's important to get treatment as soon as possible for this, and any other, STD.

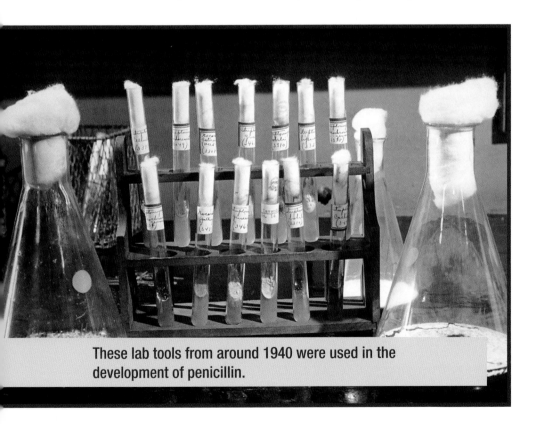

These lab tools from around 1940 were used in the development of penicillin.

Because of penicillin, many of the symptoms of syphilis—especially in its last and most advanced stage—are uncommon in developed western nations today. They still exist in the developing world, where people do not have easy access to proper screening, treatment, or supplies. Providing access to testing and treatment to people around the world may help to truly eradicate syphilis in the future.

## HOW DOES IT SPREAD?

From ancient history to today, there's still only one main way to contract and spread syphilis—sex. While it can occasionally be acquired by nonsexual means, that's uncommon. For example, cases where someone has gotten the disease from kissing an infected person are not entirely unheard of, but they are still rare. This requires actual contact with an active sore on or in the infected person's mouth and an abrasion or cut on the other person.

The *Treponema pallidum* bacterium needs moisture to survive and thrive. That is why its main mode of transmission between individuals is through sexual contact, specifically vaginal, anal, or oral sex. Another way it spreads is from an infected pregnant mother to her unborn child. Intravenous (IV) drug users could also potentially catch syphilis by sharing needles, but this method of transmission is relatively low and not as risky as sexual contact. However, drug users could contract HIV from sharing needles, and HIV could increase a person's risk of becoming severely ill with syphilis.

Syphilis is not spread through casual contact.

You cannot get it by sharing a meal or a drink with someone or by using the same utensils. You can't get it from shared bathtubs, showers, pools, or toilets. It's not airborne, like the viruses responsible for the flu or COVID-19. You cannot transfer it to another person via a doorknob or by sharing clothing. Knowing how syphilis spreads can help you make the best decisions for yourself as you interact with people. It makes it even more important to get tested for STDs and require your partner to also get tested before you have sex.

## STDS DON'T DISCRIMINATE

In history, certain ethnic groups, religions, and countries would blame others for the spread of syphilis. But like other STDs, syphilis does not discriminate. Whatever your sexual orientation, ethnicity, or social class is, you can contract syphilis simply because you're human. Inaccurate ideas of who is prone to syphilis, and who is not, only serve to give people a false—and dangerous—sense of security in the face of this serious disease. It also leads to unfair discrimination.

Some groups do suffer more than others from syphilis, however. Primary and secondary syphilis are found more in men than in women. Biological males who have sex with other biological males contract syphilis at higher rates than males who have sex with females only. Despite a lower percentage of new female cases recently, women cannot let their guard down either. Women tend to experience milder symptoms than men and are thus more likely to mistake syphilis for something else or to remain asymptomatic. Although they make up only around 12 percent of the U.S. population, more than 30 percent of STDs including chlamydia, gonorrhea, and syphilis were among non-Hispanic Black Americans in 2019.

Although certain groups contract syphilis at higher rates, it's wrong and inaccurate to blame any particular group of people for syphilis. Rather, we can look at the inequities in heath care and sexual education in communities who suffer from higher rates. By addressing those inequities and providing resources and education, people from more at-risk communities can be empowered to get the preventative tools, testing, and treatment that they need.

Even if you aren't part of a high-risk group, you can still contract an STD like syphilis, after just one sexual encounter with one person. The only way to be safe is to take the necessary precautions against syphilis.

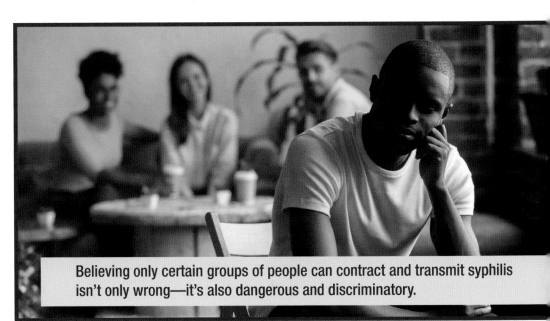

Believing only certain groups of people can contract and transmit syphilis isn't only wrong—it's also dangerous and discriminatory.

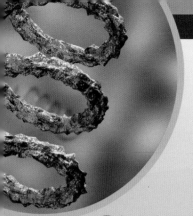

# CHAPTER 2

# STAGES AND SYMPTOMS OF SYPHILIS

Syphilis occurs in stages, with different symptoms at each stage. While a person might think syphilis is no big deal in the early stage, they still need to get treatment so it doesn't progress to secondary or tertiary syphilis. Syphilis in early stages can still be cured, while the damage caused in later stages can only be treated. It might take anywhere between 10 and 90 days for the first symptoms of primary syphilis to begin. From there, it may take weeks or months to develop secondary syphilis symptoms, and 10 to 30 years to develop tertiary syphilis symptoms, which are deadly. Recognizing the symptoms of syphilis can help people catch it in the earliest stage and cure it.

# PRIMARY SYPHILIS SYMPTOMS

The first stage of syphilis, called primary syphilis, occurs soon after sexual contact with an infected person. The main symptom of primary syphilis is a sore called a chancre. A chancre is an open sore that has a firm base. Chancre sores occur at the point of contact where the infection first affects the person receiving it. Almost always, chancres are painless. Sufferers may not even notice they have developed them.

In biological females, chancre sores can develop on the outside or inside of the vagina or on the cervix, directly above the vagina. Even prominent, exterior sores might not be immediately visible or noticeable. Sometimes, chancres might be hidden in the folds of the labia.

Biological males with primary syphilis may get chancres on the penis, anus, and rectum. These can remain unnoticed when developing in certain areas, such as the folds of the foreskin of the penis, under the

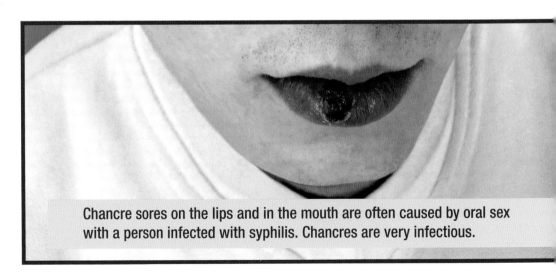

Chancre sores on the lips and in the mouth are often caused by oral sex with a person infected with syphilis. Chancres are very infectious.

scrotum, or at the base of the penis.

No matter a person's anatomical sex, chancre sores can also occur on the mouth, lips, or tongue, and sometimes even on the hands or eyes. Exposure in this area of the body is most likely when someone engages in oral sex with an infected person with an active sore

# A CASE OF MISTAKEN IDENTITY

Syphilis chancres may be confused with "canker" sores because of the similarity of their names. And canker sores can be confused with cold sores because they seem similar in many ways. Cold sores carry the herpes simplex virus. They are painful blisters that occur usually outside of the mouth on the lips. Canker sores are white or gray sores that occur in the mouth. Cold sores and canker sores can be irritating and painful, but both are relatively harmless. Meanwhile, the painless syphilis chancre is anything but harmless. You might go months or even years without detection, all while syphilis is spreading in your body.

Because of its common symptoms, syphilis has been and is still often mistaken for other ailments including herpes, measles, typhus, smallpox, fungal infections, leprosy, and dozens of other infections. It's also mistaken for everyday health issues, such as ingrown hairs, acne, and minor injuries. Because of that, it has sometimes been known as the "great imitator" or the "great pretender." It can be overlooked because, unlike other bacterial infections like gonorrhea, there is no burning or discharge. The confusion over syphilis symptoms and terms makes it even more important to talk to a medical professional as soon as you think you might have it.

on the genitals.

Each open, reddish chancre sore is painless, round or oval, and firm. It is relatively clean, with no pus or discharge. It can be easily overlooked. If you get one, it will typically appear as early as two weeks or as late as ten or more weeks after exposure. These lesions, without being treated, typically go away within about three to six weeks.

Another symptom affects the lymph nodes (oval-shaped organs that are part of the human immune system) in the groin and inner thighs. These may swell, harden, and become tender. If primary syphilis isn't treated, it will progress to the secondary stage.

## SECONDARY SYPHILIS SYMPTOMS

The progression through the stages of syphilis is different for every person. The stages can last for weeks, months, or years. The progression from primary to secondary syphilis is marked by the bacterium spreading through the body. The bacterial infection travels through your blood, entering your skin cells, liver, and joints. It also affects the lymphatic system, the muscles, and the brain.

When the chancres from the first stage have healed, they are often followed by a rash that arises about six weeks to three months later. These rashes most commonly occur on the palms or the soles of the feet. Lesions can also occur on the trunk of the body, such as the back and chest. Usually, the rash doesn't itch, as some rashes tend to. At the same time, chancres may develop in one's mouth or throat and even deeper

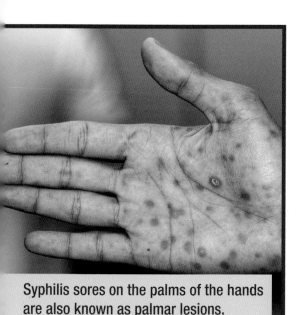

Syphilis sores on the palms of the hands are also known as palmar lesions.

within the body, on one's bones and internal organs.

During the secondary stage, syphilis can be extremely contagious. Bacteria are secreted by the chancres and can easily spread, especially through sexual activity. Other symptoms might cause some real discomfort. People with syphilis may have sore throats or headaches, develop a fever, or experience aches and joint pains. Some people even lose some of their hair.

Some people don't develop noticeable symptoms in this stage of syphilis. This may seem like a good thing, but it can keep people from getting the diagnosis they need to get treatment. The symptoms of secondary syphilis could subside and disappear in a couple of weeks. Others have these symptoms recur over the course of months, even a year. If a person doesn't treat secondary syphilis, it can turn into tertiary syphilis, which can be fatal.

## SILENT SYPHILIS: THE LATENT STAGE

Between the symptoms of secondary syphilis and tertiary syphilis, there is often a time when there are no symptoms at all. This is called the latent stage, or latency. Latent means "hidden" or "concealed." People might think they're healed. But this does not mean that symptoms will not return. Some researchers don't consider this a true stage of the disease, since there are no symptoms.

Some people's latent stage lasts months or years. Some carriers may go 10 to 30 years without significant symptoms. This can keep people from getting the treatment they need to stop syphilis in its tracks. Without treatment, secondary syphilis may progress to the final stage—tertiary syphilis.

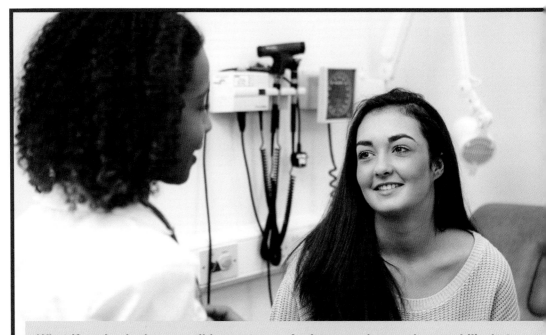

What if you've had some mild symptoms of primary and secondary syphilis, but those went away? You may just be in the latent stage, and it's very important you get tested and treated before the disease progresses.

# TERTIARY SYPHILIS SYMPTOMS

Tertiary syphilis, or late syphilis, occurs after latency. This stage presents the most advanced, frightening, and dangerous health problems. The patient will likely not be contagious anymore, but the effects of the infection can be fatal.

In the tertiary stage, *Treponema pallidum* reactivates and begins to multiply. Syphilis begins to spread through much of the body. The bones and joints are affected, as well as the eyes. Blindness is a common symptom of this late stage. Even more important, organ systems are affected, including the nervous system and circulatory system. The symptoms in this stage depend on which organ system the bacterium has affected.

Sufferers of later-stage syphilis can develop gummas—tumors or large growths (granulomas) that are nonmalignant (non-cancerous) but can be large and rubbery. These are actually a reaction of the human immune system in a last-ditch effort to fight off syphilis. In this case, the tissues grow to block or slow down the progress of the bacteria. They can occur anywhere in the body, both internally and at the surface of the skin. Syphilitic gummas commonly affect a person's joints when they grow on the skeleton. They often form on the leg, below the knee. When they grow inside the body—for example, on the liver—they may affect organ functions. Other effects are bone and joint pain from the inflammation.

One of systems that can be harmed by tertiary syphilis is the cardiovascular system, including the blood vessels and main arteries. Syphilis causes narrowing of the blood vessels. This may lead to chest pain and may eventually cause a heart attack, possibly a fatal one. The most important artery leading from the heart to the abdomen, the aorta, is also affected. The muscular and elastic tissue that helps pump blood in the body becomes inflamed. This inflammation weakens that tissue, leaving it less able to do its job. The same is true for the heart valves that open and close to pump blood. Failure of the heart valves leads to heart failure and death. A weakened aorta can lead to a heart murmur. It can even rupture, an event called an aortic aneurysm, which can be fatal.

# NEUROLOGICAL SYMPTOMS IN LATE-STAGE SYPHILIS

Neurosyphilis occurs when the disease causes deterioration, or breaking down, of the human nervous system, especially the brain and spinal cord. While relatively rare, it remains a possibility for those who leave syphilis untreated. There are several categories of neurosyphilis, which depend on the severity and extent of the infection. It mostly afflicts those in the tertiary stage. As the CDC warns, however, it can occur at any stage of syphilis infection. It can cause headaches and sensory issues. It can also cause trouble with coordinating muscle movements and even paralysis.

Meningovascular neurosyphilis—sometimes known as meningeal neurosyphilis—generally occurs in the late stage, though it can also develop in someone who has recently been infected, either within the first few months or within years of exposure. Nausea, vomiting, a stiff

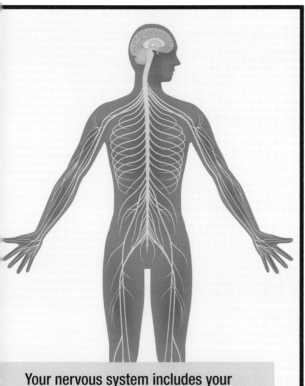

Your nervous system includes your brain, spinal cord, and all the nerves in your body. It allows you to think, move, regulate bodily functions, and more. If syphilis spreads to the nervous system, many complications can arise.

neck, and headaches are typical symptoms. Loss of vision and hearing can occur, too. Its name derives from the meninges, the membranes that cover the central nervous system, which it inflames, along with the small blood vessels in the brain itself.

Some people with neurosyphilis develop general paresis. It is rare these days in developed nations, but it was a fearsome and widespread condition in the past, when it was known as GPI—"general paresis of the insane" or "general paralysis of the insane." People with GPI were known to have grand delusions, forgetfulness, and strange behavior. This can be confused with other mental disorders and may include noticeable mental impairment. The person may seem "off" in some way, experiencing mood swings or sharp shifts in personality. Memory problems and disorientation can occur, as well as depression. In advanced cases, a person might have chronic dementia and even hallucinations. This is one reason that some people confuse it for Alzheimer's disease. General paresis can take anywhere from three to 30 years to arise. Penicillin is prescribed in treating it, but, as with the other late-stage syphilitic symptoms, the antibiotic can only beat back the infection; it cannot reverse the damage already done.

People with neurosyphilis may also develop tabes dorsalis, or syphilitic myelopathy. In these cases, syphilis damages the nerves in the spinal cord, which compromises the sensory signals a person receives from the surrounding world. The earliest symptoms are sharp and sudden pains in the legs. Other signs are a sense of tingling, burning, or coldness in the lower half of the body. This particular complication of syphilis brings with it poor balance and coordination, which can cause trouble with walking and other common movements. Called sensory ataxia, this condition comes from being unable to judge one's position in relation to the ground. People with ataxia find it hard to walk in a straight line or over uneven surfaces. They also have difficulty navigating sudden turns. Victims' feet may become less sensitive to stimuli and temperature changes, becoming numb. Ulcers may also develop on the feet. Other effects of tabes dorsalis that are nerve-related are problems with vision, hearing, and a loss of control of bladder and bowel movements. At this advanced stage, a person might regain some health with proper treatment but usually won't return to normal health.

# MYTHS AND FACTS

## MYTH
Syphilis is a slow death sentence.

## FACT
Syphilis is completely curable when treated in its early stages, and it's treatable in later stages. Some people experience few symptoms.

## MYTH
Syphilis only affects the genitals because it's a sexually transmitted disease.

## FACT
While chancre sores in the primary stage of syphilis may be found on the genitals, syphilis can spread to affect many different organ systems and body parts.

## MYTH
Syphilis is a disease of the past.

## FACT
While today's treatment is more effective than treatments in previous times, syphilis still exists and you can still contract it through risky sexual behaviors.

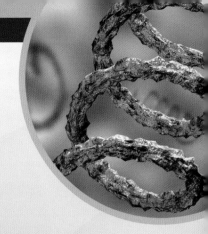

# CHAPTER 3

# GETTING TESTED FOR *SYPHILIS*

Syphilis often mimics other diseases and disorders with its symptoms. Sometimes symptoms are so mild people might not realize that they have it. That's why it's even more important to get tested for syphilis if you have any of the symptoms or have had sex with someone who might be infected. As with other STDs, it takes only one sexual encounter to get infected. Getting tested can give you peace of mind if it's negative or a plan for treatment if it's positive. You can also keep your sexual partner safe by letting them know your results as soon as you find out.

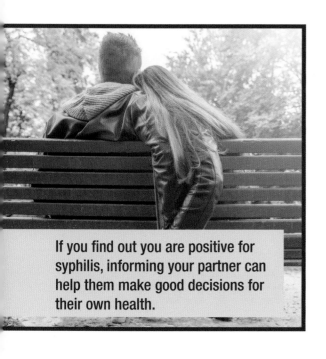

If you find out you are positive for syphilis, informing your partner can help them make good decisions for their own health.

## WHO SHOULD BE TESTED?

If you have syphilis symptoms and may have had sex with someone who could be infected, you should get a test. That includes sex with someone you're in a monogamous relationship with but who hasn't been recently tested for STDs after they had sex with someone else.

Some people are at a higher risk of contracting syphilis, and they should get tested more regularly. This includes people who have multiple sex partners, a partner who has multiple sex partners, and people who have sex without a condom. Other risk factors include having HIV, AIDS, or another STD, such as gonorrhea. Biological men who have sex with other biological men should be tested for STDs, such as syphilis, regularly. Women should also be tested if they find out they're pregnant, because syphilis can be passed to an unborn baby and cause complications and even death.

## WHERE CAN I BE TESTED?

You can get tested for syphilis and other STDs at a doctor's office or a health clinic specializing in STD screenings and treatment. There are several pros and cons as to which course might be best.

You may feel comfortable with a doctor you already know and trust. On the other hand, you may feel uncomfortable talking to your family doctor or pediatrician about sexual health if they've known you since childhood. It's also possible that your primary care doctor doesn't provide the necessary tests in their office. Still, they will be able to direct you to a place that can do the test. And even if you feel awkward discussing sex with your doctor, remember that they should only have your health in mind and shouldn't judge you.

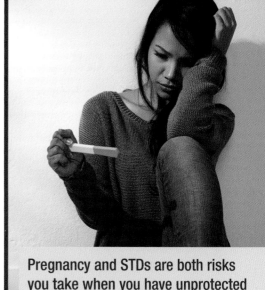

Pregnancy and STDs are both risks you take when you have unprotected sex. STDs like syphilis can also complicate pregnancy, which is why it's important to be tested if you find out you're pregnant.

You can also get tested at an STD clinic. These tests may be cheaper, especially if your state, county, or locality funds low-income health services. Many organizations also offer counseling geared especially at adolescents and young people. Another group that offers similar services is Planned Parenthood.

Consult the internet or other listings for the closest local resources. Those offering both screening and treatment are best. Make sure to plan accordingly. For example, low-cost or free clinics might have irregular hours or long waits for their affordable care so you might have to be flexible with your schedule.

# TYPES OF SYPHILIS TESTS

Some people feel nervous about going for a test for STDs, including syphilis. It can help to know what to expect from the test. The slight social discomfort of requesting a syphilis screening or the mild physical discomfort of bloodwork are minor compared to the risks of living with untreated syphilis. In this case, what you don't know can hurt you.

There are several different types of tests for syphilis. Common tests are rapid plasma reagin (RPR) tests and venereal disease research laboratory (VDRL) tests. Both tests look for antibodies to the syphilis bacterium, which are proteins made by the immune system to fight the disease. Both of these screening tests can be done with a blood sample, and VDRL can also be done on spinal fluid if the disease is in its advanced stage.

Diagnosing syphilis requires two steps. The first is meant to detect that a syphilis infection is a definite possibility. If the first step results in a positive, then the second step is a more specific diagnostic test. The initial step—using RPR or VDRL tests—does not test directly for syphilis. Instead, it tests for syphilis antibodies in the blood. Antibodies are protein molecules the body creates to fight diseases, including infections caused by bacteria and viruses. The human body makes antibodies that respond to syphilis, but similar ones also arise when someone has Lyme disease, certain kinds of pneumonia, malaria, and other

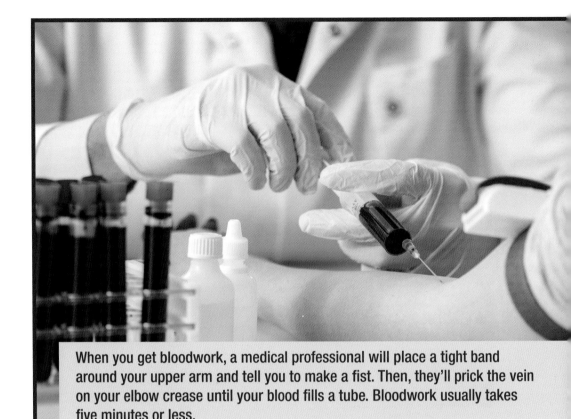

When you get bloodwork, a medical professional will place a tight band around your upper arm and tell you to make a fist. Then, they'll prick the vein on your elbow crease until your blood fills a tube. Bloodwork usually takes five minutes or less.

conditions, like tuberculosis and lupus. Since these tests may result in false positives due to these other conditions, it's called nontreponemal (or it doesn't prove the existence of *Treponema pallidum*, the bacterium that causes syphilis).

A second set of tests further confirms a syphilis infection. These treponemal (more able to show the existence of syphilis) tests are less likely to turn up false positives because of other conditions a person has. They do have one weakness, though. They test only whether someone has at some point been infected.

This means they will still yield false positives if the person being tested has been cured of syphilis. Tests that look for syphilis bacteria and not just the antibodies can only be done in specialized labs. If your test comes back negative, you will know that you don't have syphilis. If your test comes back positive, you can get treatment for it right away.

## TREPONEMAL TESTS

Treponemal tests might be ordered after the nontreponemal tests return positive. These are less common, but they test directly for syphilis bacteria. Treponemal tests include darkfield microscopy, in which a chancre sore is scraped and then the samples are placed on a slide and viewed through a microscope. Samples can also be taken from affected lymph nodes. If the darkfield test comes out positive, doctors can be almost certain that someone has syphilis in one of its stages.

Another process that can confirm the presence of syphilis is molecular testing. This test looks for genetic material of the bacteria from a blood or spinal fluid sample. It's useful for detecting primary syphilis, secondary syphilis, and congenital syphilis, especially when dark field microscopy isn't available.

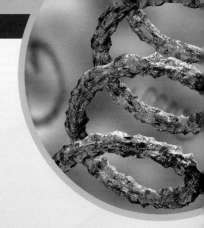

# CHAPTER 4

# TREATMENT AND SUPPORT

Finding out you've tested positive for syphilis can be stressful and overwhelming. No one goes into sex expecting to get an STD, so your diagnosis can come as a shock. Even though you might have big feelings around your diagnosis, it's important to take action and get treatment. Likely, your doctor or the clinic that tested you will offer you a course of treatment. If you discover your infection early on, the resources are out there to help you overcome syphilis and have a complete recovery. Accepting this treatment and any support you need will help you take back control over your sexual health.

# PRESCRIBING PENICILLIN

Penicillin was the first drug to completely cure syphilis infections, and it's still the top choice for doctors to prescribe today. Also used for other bacterial conditions like ear infections, a single dose of penicillin often cures syphilis if the infection has occurred within the last year. The type of penicillin used for syphilis is benzathine benzylpenicillin, which is also used for pneumonia, meningitis, and other ailments.

Penicillin cures syphilis in the primary stage. Sometimes it's given to patients with a shot, often injected directly into the muscles of the buttocks (intramuscularly). Other times, it's provided intravenously—that is, through a needle into the bloodstream. Unlike other antibiotics, unfortunately, penicillin does not seem to be effective when taken orally, in pill form. That means treatment won't be as simple as taking a pill, but it will be very effective.

Patients allergic to penicillin must be extra careful. Doctors will first try to desensitize an allergic patient to penicillin slowly, especially if they feel that the symptoms are minor compared to the effectiveness of penicillin as a syphilis cure. Severe allergies prevent easy desensitization, so alternative antibiotics such as doxycycline, tetracycline, ceftriaxone, or azithromycin may be prescribed. These have been shown to be adequate for the first and second stages. But nothing quite substitutes for penicillin in a late-stage patient. It's important for you to tell a doctor if you have any drug allergies or a history of antibiotic reactions before they treat you. That will help them weigh benefits and risks, and come up with the safest plan for your treatment.

Even if you don't have an allergy to penicillin, you may have a reaction to it that includes a rash, joint and muscle aches, headaches, chills, and a fever. This is called a Jarisch-Herxheimer reaction. This should clean up in a day or so, and it's common. If you have any lingering side effects of penicillin, you should tell your doctor.

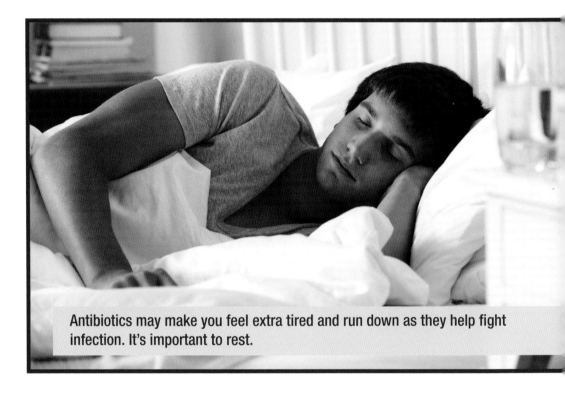

Antibiotics may make you feel extra tired and run down as they help fight infection. It's important to rest.

After treatment, doctors will usually require that you come in for at least two follow-up blood tests, around six months and a year after your initial treatment. This is to make sure that the treatment has been effective. With early detection and proper treatment, you should be cured.

# CAN I GET A VACCINE?

Vaccines can help greatly decrease the number of people who contract a disease. A vaccine activates your immune system to produce antibodies to a disease. This helps your body learn how to fight the disease before you contract it. Most vaccines contain a killed or weakened germ that doesn't make you sick but does help make you immune to the disease.

Currently, there's no vaccine for syphilis. That's because penicillin has had staying power when it comes to fighting this disease. Other bacterial STDs, like gonorrhea, have developed strains in recent years with increased resistance to antibiotics. Resistant strains might demand larger doses, although it's a delicate balancing act because using antibiotics carelessly can cause unexpectedly strong, newer strains of diseases to arise in human populations. The continuing effectiveness of penicillin has made the creation of a syphilis vaccine a low priority for the medical field.

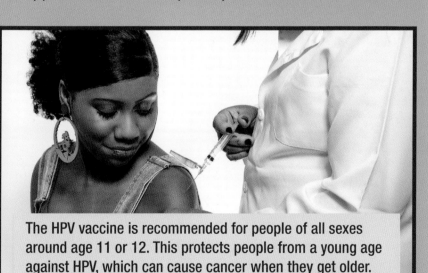

The HPV vaccine is recommended for people of all sexes around age 11 or 12. This protects people from a young age against HPV, which can cause cancer when they get older.

However, there are vaccines for other STDs, which you should consider if you're sexually active. HPV is the most common STD, and it has more than 100 strains. Some of the strains can cause cancer if left untreated. Fortunately, there's an effective vaccine for HPV, which you can receive right in your doctor's office. Vaccines are also available for hepatitis A and hepatitis B, which can be contracted through sex.

# TREATING LATE-STAGE SYPHILIS

Usually all you need to treat primary, secondary, and latent syphilis is a single injection of penicillin. That is often enough to kill off all the bacteria in your body. However, people with tertiary syphilis need a different plan for treatment. While antibiotics can help treat the infection, they can't undo the damage that's already been done to organs and body parts.

Many patients with late latent syphilis or tertiary syphilis are treated with one weekly dose of penicillin for three weeks. Still others, further down the road into tertiary syphilis, especially neurosyphilis, need more penicillin. This is because they have more of the syphilis-causing bacteria in their bodies and probably in a variety of organ systems. They may receive penicillin every few hours or every day for a recommended number of days.

Other antibiotics, such as ceftriaxone, may be attempted if someone is truly allergic and has a more serious late-stage form of syphilis. Unfortunately, penicillin is still the only truly effective treatment for neurosyphilis and other late-stage symptoms. With proper treatment and care, a person's health may improve greatly.

## COMPLICATIONS OF CONGENITAL SYPHILIS

A person who is pregnant or intends to someday be pregnant needs to get treatment for syphilis fast—for their own sake and that of their future child. Syphilis can spread from a pregnant mother to a child in the womb, with possibly terrible results. This is called congenital syphilis. The bacteria are usually transferred via the placenta, which connects the fetus to the uterus. If not earlier, getting a syphilis screening upon learning you are pregnant is crucial to protecting you and your baby. The National Institutes of Health estimate that 50

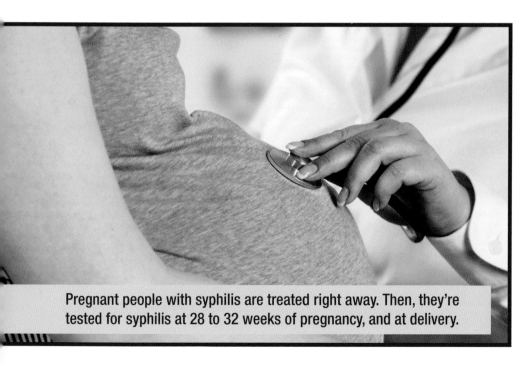

Pregnant people with syphilis are treated right away. Then, they're tested for syphilis at 28 to 32 weeks of pregnancy, and at delivery.

percent of children that contract syphilis before birth die in the womb or shortly after being born. Other babies may have a physical deformity called "saddle nose" — they are missing the bridge of the nose most people are born with.

Newborns with congenital syphilis may suffer from fever or unusual irritability, failure to gain weight or thrive (grow and develop properly), or rashes on the face, mouth, anus, and genitals. Infants sometimes discharge mucus, pus, and/or bloody discharge from the nose. These early symptoms are considered early congenital syphilis and manifest in the first three months of a child's life.

The majority of infected children are asymptomatic at birth but develop late congenital syphilis after about two years of life. Sadly, these very young children can experience similar symptoms to adults entering their tertiary stage of infection, like paresis and tabes dorsalis.

They may also have their own unique symptoms. Among these are Hutchinson teeth, which have an unusual notched and pegged appearance. Other problems include eye disorders, impaired hearing or deafness, bone pain and malformed arms or legs, and gray patches and skin scarring in the groin area. Infected women who receive penicillin treatment early in their pregnancy greatly reduce the chance of their baby developing congenital syphilis. If you're pregnant or ever thinking of becoming pregnant, deciding to get treatment can not only save your life, but that of your baby.

# THE DEADLY HIV/SYPHILIS COMBINATION

HIV is a virus that attacks the immune system. This keeps people from being able to fight disease and infection. If untreated, HIV can turn into AIDs, which can be fatal.

Syphilis is already a dangerous disease. But if you also have HIV, the dangers dramatically increase. Syphilis itself can increase the chances of catching HIV. That is because active sores act as open doors for HIV. The CDC estimates that someone having sexual contact with an HIV-infected person has two to five times a greater risk of contracting HIV when syphilis is present.

Once infected, carrying both HIV and syphilis at the same time is even more dangerous. Even effective treatments in recent years have not curbed its deadly effects in many patients. While syphilis may or may not advance through to the tertiary stage on its own, HIV attacks the immune system so badly that syphilis often does far worse damage than it ordinarily would. In many cases, HIV speeds up the spread of syphilis throughout the body.

Having both HIV and syphilis together is a particular concern for biological males who have sex with other biological males. An average of four in 10 males who have sex with males are infected with HIV. And the stigma around homosexuality may keep people who need treatment from receiving it.

# 10 GREAT QUESTIONS
## TO ASK A DOCTOR

**1** How often should I be tested for STDs?

**2** What are some ways I can prevent syphilis?

**3** What are my risk factors for contracting syphilis?

**4** Do I have to tell my previous sexual partners if I have a positive diagnosis?

**5** What are my options for treatment?

**6** What stage of syphilis am I in?

**7** Will there be any lasting effects from syphilis after treatment?

**8** When will I no longer be contagious?

**9** What precautions should I take after treatment?

**10** Are there any local support groups for teens with STDs?

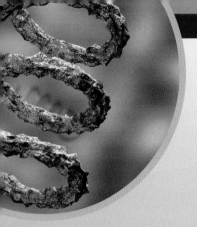

CHAPTER 5

# STAYING SMART ABOUT SYPHILIS

**M**aybe you don't have an STD, but you want to learn how to stay smart about sex to prevent them. Fortunately, there are many things you can do to reduce your chances of contracting syphilis. Communication, protection, and education can go a long way in keeping you safe from sexually transmitted diseases.

Since syphilis is transmitted primarily through vaginal, anal, and oral sex, the most effective way to keep from contracting it is to not have sex. This is called abstinence, and it's a choice that many teens make for many different reasons. However, if you do choose to have sex, there are many ways for you to minimize your risk of contracting syphilis.

# REDUCING RISK

Sex can be risky business, but your level of risk is dependent on the precautions you take. While syphilis will not infect any particular kind of person more readily than another, there are lifestyle and behavior choices that can put you at greater risk of being infected—with syphilis and a host of other STDs, both viral and bacterial.

Having multiple sexual partners in a short span of time, or dating several partners at once, puts someone at greater risk of syphilis exposure. Other behaviors can indirectly put you in situations that make you more vulnerable. For example, underage binge drinking and substance abuse can impair a young person's judgment with sex. Having one STD can open you up to others, as you can see with the link between HIV

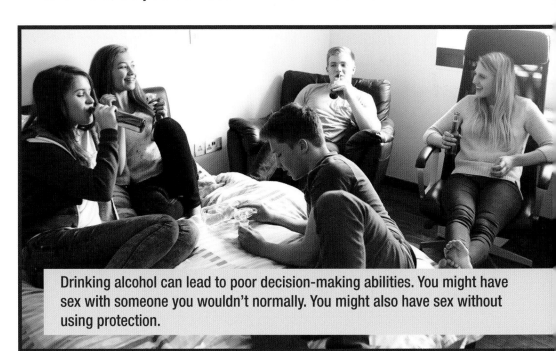

Drinking alcohol can lead to poor decision-making abilities. You might have sex with someone you wouldn't normally. You might also have sex without using protection.

and syphilis. Not using condoms, or not using them consistently or correctly, greatly increases your risk of contracting an STD. Ask yourself if you fall into any of these risk factors, and what you can do to make your behavior safer and smarter.

# COMMUNICATION MAKES A DIFFERENCE

If you're in a sexual relationship with someone, communication is key. You need to let your partner know if you've had sex with other people and if you've been tested for STDs after those encounters. You definitely have to let them know if you have an active STD or STI. And you need to trust that your partner is also being honest with you about their sexual history and testing history.

Conversations like this may seem like they're the opposite of fun and spontaneous. However, they'll go a long way in keeping you and your partner healthy. Choose a time to talk about this when you have enough time and space to have a real conversation. Talk about it before you start having sex, so you know what precautions to take.

You and your partner will also need to talk about protection. Being monogamous, getting tested regularly, and using protection (condoms) are steps that can keep you safe from STDs. There are several types of protection you can use. There's the external condom (also called the male condom), that is worn over an erect penis. There's also an internal condom (also called a female condom) that is worn inside the vagina or anus. For oral sex, you can use a dental dam, which you can buy online. You can also make a dental dam yourself by cutting the tip off an external condom and cutting up one side to make a flat sheet. Place that over the genitals or anus before oral sex to create a barrier.

Condoms are incredibly effective against STDs. When used correctly every time you have sex, they are 98 percent effective against most STIs, such as gonorrhea and chlamydia. While they reduce your risk for syphilis, there's still a chance you can contract or transmit the disease while using a condom because syphilis can be spread skin-to-skin. If a chancre is anywhere that the condom isn't covering, the disease can still be spread. Remember that even one sex act with an infected person can lead to an STD if you don't use protection. That means you and your partner need to be committed to using condoms every single time you have any form of sex.

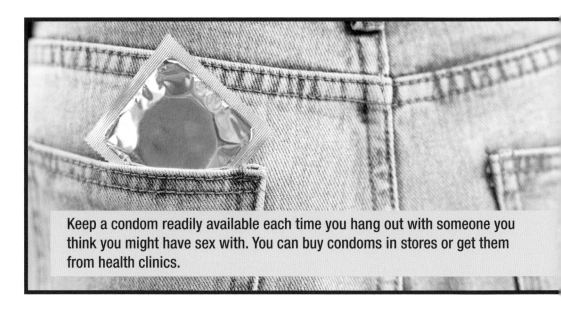

Keep a condom readily available each time you hang out with someone you think you might have sex with. You can buy condoms in stores or get them from health clinics.

# HAVING "THE TALK"

If you test positive for an STD, you have to have a very serious conversation with your sexual partner. It may be hard to summon the courage. You may still be reeling from the news. You may not know how you were infected, and you may wonder if you gave it to your partner or if they gave it to you. Nevertheless, you owe it to yourself and your partner to be honest and straightforward about your condition. It may be uncomfortable and embarrassing. You might be worried your partner's reaction to the news. But you will be saving them pain and discomfort later on. The sooner they get tested, the sooner your lives can go back to normal.

You might need to educate your partner on what your diagnosis means. Be prepared for possible concern from your partner. Arm yourself with knowledge about how syphilis is and isn't spread. This will reassure the person that you know what you are doing, and your confidence and honesty will shine through. Often, having this conversation may show you how much your partner cares about you. You may be pleasantly surprised: a quality partner will be open-minded and willing to work with you. You can decide together what precautions to take. For example, someone with an active flare-up, especially early syphilis, may want to avoid even kissing someone because an open sore inside the mouth could be dangerous.

It's also important to talk to former partners about a diagnosis. They might be someone you don't communicate with anymore. However, knowing that you've kept someone safe and stopped the spread of syphilis will hopefully be a relief.

# STAY SMART ONLINE

The internet can be a great source of information about STD prevention, symptoms, and treatment. Looking up reputable websites (like those of the CDC or National Institutes of Health) is a good start when researching syphilis. The internet can also help you find clinics and support. Online advice and information about syphilis should be approached with caution, however. Not all of it will be correct or properly vetted by professionals. Look for websites that end in .gov, .edu, or .org to make sure they're accurate, or read articles that are written by medical doctors. That'll help you get the best information possible.

Be equally careful when it comes to online support groups, comment threads, and social media pages. While some are helpful and perform an invaluable service—especially for those who are looking for someone to relate to in the middle of an STD scare—always protect your identity and your privacy. Report anyone who asks for money or makes unusual requests. Never give personal information, and let a trusted adult know if someone is making you uncomfortable online.

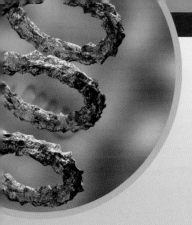

# CHAPTER 6

# COPING AND MOVING FORWARD

**S**yphilis can affect your physical health and also your mental health. Any STD diagnosis can make a person feel out of control and full of emotions. You can use coping tools to deal with your diagnosis and any concerns around your relationships and reputation. After you deal with your physical treatment for syphilis and take care of your mental health, you may feel even stronger and more capable of dealing with difficult situations. This can help you move forward and make the best choices for you and your future.

# EMBARRASSMENT AND SHAME

When people find out they have syphilis, they may feel embarrassment and even shame. Embarrassment means feeling that you did something bad or wrong. Shame takes it a step further. It means feeling that you *are* bad or wrong. These thoughts and feelings are natural, but they can also have a serious impact on your self-esteem and mental well-being.

STDs can really rock your self-esteem. Even if you have an STD, you are worthy of compassion and care—from yourself and others.

Stigmas around sex can lead someone to feel shame. Sex is often an awkward, or even taboo, topic of discussion to begin with, especially between young people and parents or other adults in authority. This embarrassment and silence surrounding sex extends to syphilis, which can seem uncommon and particularly "bad." A herpes sore on the mouth may be considered normal, with about half of Americans carrying HSV-1, or oral herpes, while a syphilis chancre is something few people would want to admit to.

At the same time, a syphilis diagnosis is something a young person takes very personally. Realizing that you are not defined by an infection may be difficult, but it's necessary for your mental health. Syphilis is something you have, not something you are. Shame is not only counterproductive; it can be harmful, too. It's another way of blaming yourself. Of course, this is another dead end: we can't change the past. All you can do is learn from what happened and make more informed choices in the future.

## THERAPY MAKES A DIFFERENCE

One of the best ways to get a handle on your mental health is to go to therapy or counseling. A mental health counselor or psychologist will listen to you without judgement and teach you coping skills for difficult situations and feelings. You can ask a parent or guardian to help you find a mental health counselor. You can also talk to your doctor about mental health resources in your area. Some counseling services are low-cost or even free with insurance. Joining a support group might also be a good option for you.

Counseling or therapy can help you get over the emotional effects of your syphilis situation and can also help you express

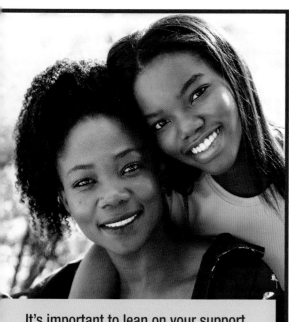

It's important to lean on your support system when you're going through a hard time, whether that's family, friends, or a combination of both.

your feelings, set goals, and develop coping skills and stress-reduction techniques. Many people benefit from the structure and guidance that these kinds of programs offer. Therapy can provide a caring and impartial listener who provides unbiased advice. They might teach you ways to feel calmer through breathing exercises, meditation, and journaling. They might help you find ways to foster positive relationships in your life and cut out negative ones. Therapy can put you in the right headspace to get better—physically and mentally.

## NEGATIVE BEHAVIORS

Many times, difficult situations lead people to negative behaviors because of poor coping skills.

A person might avoid getting help or treatment. They may allow their shame to keep them from getting the support they need. They may try to forget about their problems through drinking, drugs, self-harm, and other risky behaviors. They may keep their emotions and issues bottled inside. Some people slip into depression, signs of which include withdrawing from social interaction and one's favorite activities. Shame can also lead to hiding one's diagnosis and cutting off necessary family, peer, and community connections. As always, it's important to reach out for help if you ever feel like harming yourself. Negative behaviors may seem like the easiest choice in the moment. But choosing positive behaviors will help you truly feel better and move forward.

## MAKE YOUR HEALTH A PRIORITY

Once you've been treated for an STD, you have to keep making your health a priority. That means staying smart about sexual protection and getting tested regularly. If you've been treated for syphilis, you must show up for regularly scheduled follow-up screenings. The first two are required, while follow-ups beyond those are highly recommended. Everyone who is sexually active should attempt to get screened at least once a year, whether or not they've had an STD.

Some people become unmotivated to keep up this annual testing schedule. Anyone who falls into any of these categories especially should not miss their yearly screening: those who have tested positive for other STDs, those who have had sex with more than one partner since the last screening, users of intravenous drugs, biological males who have sex with males, people who are pregnant or planning on becoming pregnant, and victims of sexual assault. Getting tested can help you catch an STD before you develop any harmful symptoms or pass it on.

## YOU HAVE THE POWER

Syphilis can seem like a death sentence. For much of history, it might have been. However, today the frightening symptoms of late-stage syphilis happen to a very small minority of those who are infected. This potentially fatal infection is also among the most treatable STDs. If you catch it early enough, you will minimize your suffering and can live out your life without having to worry about it again. But it all starts with you deciding to get screened regularly, to take serious measures to prevent infection, and to request that partners take the same precautions out of respect for you.

Rather than being a source of shame and despair, syphilis can serve as a wake-up call to reevaluate and change risky behavior. This can help someone who has recovered from getting reinfected with syphilis or contracting another STD. You can make this into a learning experience. This knowledge will give you the power you need to keep yourself and those you love safe from syphilis in the future. You can educate and support others to empower them too. Syphilis doesn't have to mean the end of your sexual health—it can be the beginning of a new, empowered chapter for you.

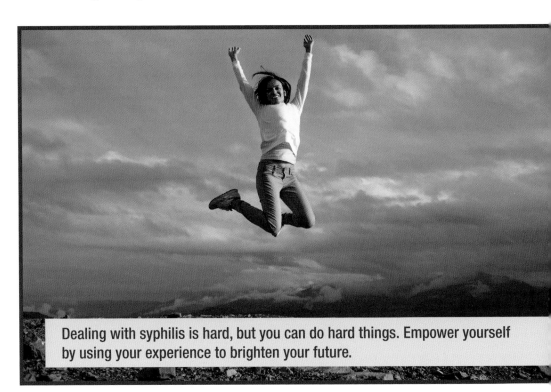

Dealing with syphilis is hard, but you can do hard things. Empower yourself by using your experience to brighten your future.

# GLOSSARY

**abstinence** The practice of abstaining from something, or not doing something that is wanted or enjoyable.

**asymptomatic** Having an infection but showing none of the common symptoms of that infection.

**brothel** A building in which prostitutes, or people paid for sex, are available.

**cervix** The constricted lower end of the female uterus, located above the vagina.

**chancre** The initial sore that appears with primary syphilis.

**congenital** Existing at or dating from birth.

**contagious** Able to spread infection or disease from one being to another.

**darkfield miscroscopy** The use of microscopes that shine a light on the object being magnified and show it against a dark background.

**dental dam** A square sheet of rubber that can be used in dentistry and oral sex.

**discrimination** Unfairly treating people unequally because of their race or beliefs.

**eradicate** To do away with completely.

**genitals** External reproductive organs.

**inequity** An instance of injustice or unfairness.

**inflammation** A response in the body to injury or illness that's marked by redness, heat, and pain.

**intramuscular** Refers to injections that are administered into a patient's muscle(s).

**intravenous** Relating to putting something into a patient's veins.

**Jarisch-Herxheimer reaction**  A set of flu-like, temporary reactions to penicillin treatments, particularly those for syphilis.

**latency**  A period in an infection's life cycle in which it appears to have disappeared and during which a patient exhibits no symptoms.

**leprosy**  An infectious disease affecting especially the skin and peripheral nerves.

**lesion**  An abnormal change in structure of an organ or part due to injury or disease.

**monogamous**  Relating to the practice of being with only one sexual partner at a time.

**nontreponemal**  Refers to an initial screening that indicates a likelihood of syphilis.

**precaution**  A measure taken beforehand to prevent harm.

**primitive**  Belonging to or characteristic of an early stage of development.

**secrete**  To form and give off.

**stigma**  A mark of shame or discredit.

**tabes dorsalis**  A particular set of symptoms of late syphilis caused by the nerves in the victim's spinal cord being damaged.

**tertiary**  The third stage or item in a series of multiple items.

**transmit**  To pass something from one person to another.

**treponemal**  Refers to secondary blood tests that confirm the presence of syphilis.

# FOR MORE INFORMATION

**Advocates for Youth**
1325 G Street NW, Suite 980
Washington, DC 20005
Website: www.advocatesforyouth.org
Instagram: @advocatesforyouth
Twitter: @AdvocatesTweets
Advocates for Youth focuses on building youth power
through sexual health and education.

**American Sexual Health Association (ASHA)**
P.O. Box 13827
Research Triangle Park, NC 27709
Website: www.ashasexualhealth.org
Instagram: @ashasexualhealth
Twitter: @InfoASHA
ASHA has worked for over 100 years to improve
the sexual health of individuals, families, and
communities through providing STD education,
support, and advocacy.

**Centers for Disease Control and Prevention**
1600 Clifton Rd
Atlanta, GA 30333
Website: www.cdc.gov
Instagram: @cdcgov
Twitter: @CDCgov
The CDC is the health protection agency of the
United States. It provides comprehensive facts and
guidance about diseases, treatment, and prevention.

**Healthy Teen Network**
1501 Saint Paul Street, Suite 114
Baltimore, MD 21202
Website: www.healthyteennetwork.org
Instagram: @healthyteennetwork
Twitter: @healthyteen
This organization works to advance social change,
    connect teens, and empower teens to protect their
    health and be more aware of sexual health issues.

**National Coalition for Sexual Health**
Website: nationalcoalitionforsexualhealth.org/contact
Instagram: @nationalcoalitionsexualhealth
Twitter: @NCSH_
This coalition works together to improve sexual health
    of Americans, make sexual health a part of normal
    conversation, and spread accurate sexual health
    information.

**Planned Parenthood**
Phone: 1-800-230-PLAN
Website: www.plannedparenthood.org
Instagram: @plannedparenthood
Twitter: @PPFA
Planned Parenthood is a nonprofit organization that
    provides sexual and reproductive health care, sexual
    education, and accurate information on sexual
    health to people around the world.

# FOR FURTHER READING

DeCarlo, Carolyn. *Everything You Need to Know About the Risks of Unprotected Sex*. New York, NY: Rosen Publishing, 2019.

Forna, Fatu, MD. *From Your Doctor to You: What Every Teenage Girl Should Know About Her Body, Sex, STDs, and Contraception.* Self-published, 2014.

Gonzales, Katheryn, and Karen Rayne PhD. *Trans+: Love, Sex, Romance, and Being You.* Washington, DC: Magination Press, 2019.

Harris, Robie H. *It's Perfectly Normal: Changing Bodies, Growing Up, Sex, Gender, and Sexual Health.* Somerville, MA: Candlewick Press, 2021.

Hope, Michelle, and Amy Lang. *The Girls' Guide to Sex Education: Over 100 Honest Answers to Urgent Questions about Puberty, Relationships, and Growing Up.* Emeryville, CA: Rockridge Press, 2018.

Moem, Erika, and Matthew Nolan. *Let's Talk About It: The Teen's Guide to Sex, Relationships, and Being a Human.* New York, NY: Random House Graphic, 2021.

Langford, Jo. *The Pride Guide: A Guide to Sexual and Social Health for LGBTQ Youth.* Lanham, MD: Rowman & Littlefield, 2018.

Parrish, Jacqueline. *Coping with Sexually Transmitted Diseases.* New York, NY: Rosen Young Adult, 2019.

Planned Parenthood. *In Case You're Curious: Questions About Sex from Young People with Answers from the Experts.* Berkeley, CA: Viva Editions, 2019.

Wolny, Philip. *I Have an STD. Now What?* New York, NY: Rosen Publishing, 2015.

# INDEX

## A

anal sex, 5, 15, 44
anus, 19, 41, 47
aorta, 25
arsenic, 13

## B

blindness, 24, 26
blood test, 4, 32, 37
blood vessels, 24, 25, 26
bones, 22, 24, 41
brain, 21, 25, 26

## C

canker sores, 20
Capone, Al, 4, 11
cardiovascular system, 24
Centers for Disease
     Control and Prevention
     (CDC), 5, 12, 25, 42,
     49
cervix, 19
chancre sores, 19, 20, 21,
     22, 28, 34, 47, 51

circulatory system, 24
Civil War, American, 12
cold sores, 20
condoms, 12, 30, 46, 47
congenital syphilis, 7, 34,
     40, 41

## D

darkfield microscopy, 34
dental dam, 47
depression, 6, 26, 53
discrimination, 16, 17

## E

eyes, 24, 41

## F

fever, 22, 37, 41

## G

Gaugin, Paul, 11
"general paresis of the
     insane" (GPI), 26, 27
genitals, 6, 21, 28, 41, 47
gonorrhea, 12, 14, 17, 20,
     30, 38, 47